From Plus-sized to Pin Up:

Mindset Strategies to Transform Your Life

Change your Mind. Change your Body.
Change your Life.

Melissa Michelle Glossup, MA, MEd

ISBN-13: 978-0692476505
ISBN-10: 0692476504

DEDICATION

To all the success stories that will be inspired by my journey and will be written to inspire others. Success does not end with your journey, it must be passed on..

CONTENTS

MELISSA MICHELLE GLOSSUP MA, MED

ACKNOWLEDGMENTS

Thank you, Dr. Mark Goulston for encouraging me to put the pen to paper and publish my story. You taught me a very important lesson in life—stop waiting. To Dr. Cruise, your skilled hand repaired a battered body and brought forth beauty and confidence. Thank you. To my family and friends who have shaped me throughout my journey; hold on, the fun is just beginning... To my mother and father, you gave your little girl the permission to dream and never taught her the mental limitations of "no" or "can't". Many people don't acknowledge dreaming is an important skill to aid success. To me, it is the foundation. Dream it. See it Be it. To Tedi, thank you for always pushing me beyond my limits and challenging me to be better. I could search the whole world over and never find someone who brings out the best in me the way you do. Love always.

PREFACE

"If you want to know what your thoughts were like yesterday, look at your body today. If you want to know what your body will be like tomorrow, look at your thoughts today."   **Navajo Proverb**

    Many people are on a constant mission to lose weight. The problem with this approach is that many dieters have conditioned themselves to FAIL. For example, the "I will start tomorrow" attitude is the first challenge to overcome. If this mindset is followed; then, tomorrow never comes and you find yourself setting next year's resolutions. In a nut shell, this is procrastination. Procrastination is not a characteristic of a successful individual. Procrastination creates a pattern of failure. Patterns become habits. Habits become actions that can make or break success. The main reason people do not succeed with any goal is that they do not put enough focus on changing the mindset toward their behavior.

Why do many people fall into this trap? The truth? *Denial.*

Many people who struggle with weight have such an emotional connection to food that they will not admit that there is a problem. This becomes apparent in many ways. One way that dieters embrace denial is that they begin to avoid the camera. I have very few photos of myself at my top weight of 375 lbs. Why? I didn't want to admit that there was a problem. I struggle with dysmorphia. What that means is by looking in the mirror, I did not see a super-morbidly obese individual. I saw someone who was a bit on the chunky side and that is about it. My perception of myself was someone around a size 14/16. I did not acknowledge that my body had ballooned into a Plus-sized 28/30. Except when I saw a picture of myself.

Through photography, I could see the naked truth about my problem, but denial would set in and I would console myself by saying that the camera adds 10 lbs. Maybe so, but a camera does not add 200 lbs. I would blame the technology instead of taking responsibility that my weight had gotten grotesquely out of control.

Interestingly enough, when I made the decision to transform my life, the first action I took was to book a professional photography session. I wanted to document my day one. It was a reminder that was a place in my life that I never wanted to revisit. For the first time, I confronted my own weakness and acknowledged that I had a problem. That was a very powerful moment for me.

I conquered 2 fears. My first fear was admitting my weight was a problem. My whole life I was afraid that someone may find out that I had a weight issue and an unhealthy relationship with food. The irony there is that I was the last one to know. Just to look at my before photos, you see someone who is totally out of control. That identity did not jive with the rest of my life. After all, I was a straight A

3

student who had completed 3 Masters degrees and worked 2 jobs, drove a new car and had a nice house and travelled often. However, in reflection, my success with school and work was also grossly out of balance. I became addicted to the success in my academic and professional life that I used being a "workaholic" to excuse my diet and exercise behaviors. I had created a life around patterns of extreme success and extreme failure.

The second fear I addressed was of being photographed. If I saw a photo of myself, I was forced to see what I had done to my body. To take that step to have my "before" picture taken changed my perception of the camera. Instead, I began using photos to track my progress. Just so you can understand, I lost 150lbs before I saw a change in the mirror. I had gone from a size 28/30 to a size 14/16. and I still saw the same reflection. Photos became a cornerstone of my success because I could SEE my progress. Being able to watch the evolution of my body, kept me motivated for what turned into a 3 and a half year process to lose 200 pounds. The remaining 35 pounds took another 3 and a half years to conquer.

To break a bad habit like yo-yo dieting, you must decide that taking control of your weight is a priority. If it isn't for any reason, you will not find success. Energy flows where your focus goes. Many people jump from diet to diet trying to find a miracle solution to a much bigger problem. Honestly, your weight and metabolism is not what you must repair. Those are the byproducts of your behaviors. Stop placing your focus on the scale and start breaking your routine. Stop grasping to empty promises of massive transformation without having to change anything about your current lifestyle or routine. Sorry, it just doesn't work that way. Once you make a decision to really change yourself; then, and only then will you will begin to see dynamic results that will last.

Success is a habit. Yes, that's right. Success is a habit. You can either build a routine that promotes success or you can follow your current routine that has landed you into a yo-yo cycle of weight loss/gain and failed diets. Every day, that becomes your choice.

"You must be the change you wish to see in the world."

Mahatma Gandhi

1

KNOW WHAT YOU WANT

"By recording your dreams and goals on paper, you set in motion the process of becoming the person you most want to be. Put your future in good hands — your own."

Mark Victor Hansen

If you just say you want to lose weight, you will probably accomplish nothing. Instead, you need to be specific about what you want to do. For example, the term "weight loss" can mean different things to different people. To be successful, you have to know what you want. I have a friend who kept telling me that she wanted to lose weight. Months passed, and nothing changed. Finally, she began working out with a trainer. At the end of her 90 day program, she had packed on 7 lbs. of muscle, lost a dress size, and looked better in a bikini than she did in her teens. She got the results she wanted because her trainer took what she said about "losing weight" and translated it into specific goals and created an action plan for success.

For my friend, "to lose weight" meant having a leaner, more muscular body was her goal. To do that, she actually had to gain weight. However, this example gives perspective to the fact that everyone has a very different, very personalized definition of success. So, what is yours?

Too often, a dieter will start a new program by identifying the total possible pounds he/she want to lose. This approach already sets the stage for failure. Why? The burden is too big. When I first began losing weight, I decided that 175 lbs. was my goal weight for a total of 200 lbs. to lose. So, when I would have a 5 or 10 pound loss, I focused on how far I still had to go. Frustrated, I would sabotage my efforts by going to the closest Starbucks to drown my dissatisfaction in 600 calories of a frozen coffee beverage with extra caramel and whip cream. (Usually more than one a day).

Every time I would get discouraged, I would gain back the 5 to 10 pounds I had lost plus 5 more. My behavior was causing my problem to get worse, not better. We are living in an age where there is an underlying expectation of instant gratification. So, if I believed my success came only after I reached my ultimate goal of 175 lbs. I was leaving too much time and opportunity for failure. This cycle became a constant disappointment, and I began to believe that I could not lose weight. My body was not the problem. My strategy was the problem.

As part of a generation defined by ADD, there was no way that I should have expected myself to stay focused on one goal for 20 months. My attention span was making me fat! Every latte, luncheon, and piece of cake would derail my determination to achieve my goal. Not because I was incapable of success, but because there was too much distance from where I was to where I wanted to be. I could not fully understand what it would be like to reach my goal. I did not know what 175 lbs. looked like. Since I could not visualize it. I could not make it real.

In a later chapter, I will illustrate how to set your weight loss goals to drive results; but for now, decide very specifically what success means for you. Do you want to be a sexy size 6? Reduce body fat and increase lean body mass? Or even become a wellness coach or a yoga instructor?

Describe how you want to look, feel, and be. What activities will you be involved in and where will you go? How will life be when you reach your goal? Write it down. Make a Vision Board. Create a clear image of your definition of success. Dream it. See it. Be it.

"When you know what you want and you want it bad enough, you'll find a way to get it." **Jim Rohn**

ACTIVITY

Pick one aspect of your life you would like to improve in your life, right now. For example, drink more water, organize your finances, or perhaps wake up 30 minutes earlier to have some me/meditation time. Whatever it is that you want to change, make it a priority.

Each week, reflect on your progress. If after seven days, you lost interest then the change was not that important to you at this time (and that is ok). Reselect another focus that is more important than the first selection and try again. When you do make progress, stick to it for 30 days. Then, decide if you want to continue with the new routine, or not. Continue to grow by adding on to the change in behavior or selecting something new to work on each month.

Keep track of your evolution over the course of a year. Choose to be faster, thinner, and more successful. Celebrate your personal growth. Create a culture of self-evolution.

NOTES

2

IDENTIFY YOUR "WHY?"

To make a permanent change in your behavior you must identify 2 things:

1) What do you want to change?

2) Why do you want to change?

To make the decision to change is good; but to fully commit yourself to that change, you must identify your "why?" The combination of understanding your "what" and your "why" will allow your rational brain to justify the change in behavior. The main reason diets fail is due to loss of motivation. When motivation is lost, it is because that "why" for the individual was not strong enough to curb the temptation to revert back to old habits.

For the first 26 years of my life, my "why" was not strong enough. As a child, I carried extra weight. I was 8 years old when I attended my first Weight Watchers class. This had a significant impact on me as I learned the vicious cycle of serial dieting at a very young age. It is interesting to look back on some of the crazy behaviors I learned. For example, do not eat before you weigh, then after the meeting go binge at your favorite restaurant. Also, make sure you went to the meetings on Friday or Saturday, so you could cheat all weekend then have 5 days to lose weight before the next weigh in. I will be honest, being exposed to such extreme behaviors had a negative impact on the relationship I had with food.

I felt isolated and alone. None of my friends had to go to monitor their food intake. I resented being overweight and I rebelled against what it was I was "supposed" to do. I began to sneak food and saved money to buy candy and soda. When I would not lose weight, or gain, I would cry and pretend like I had no idea why. My biggest fear was that my classmates would find out I was a member of Weight Watchers. During that time, there were few overweight kids, so I was being teased, anyway, so I did not want another reason to stand out for being different.

When I was 16, after several failed attempts at Weight Watchers, I had reached 205 lbs. My mother enrolled me in a program called Metabolic Research Center. Basically, it was a high protein, low carb diet that monitored PH levels in the body to make sure you maintained a state of ketosis, or fat burning. To make the diet simple, they had bars and shakes to simplify the daily menu. The also had protein supplements that you were supposed to take in between meals. I was fully repulsed by the taste of these and for a short time became bulimic.

I did find weight loss success during my time on this program, but it was due more from refusing to eat and getting sick on their supplements. Old habits die hard. After each weigh in, I would convince my mother to take me to my favorite restaurant where I would consume soup, salad, rolls, chopped steak with onions, a baked potato, and either pecan pie or cheese cake. Then, I would not eat for the next 6 days. Yet, I was losing weight, getting attention from boys, and even competed in a beauty pageant.

During my senior year when I turned 18, we decided that the cost of staying on the program was too much (around $400 per month); so, my parents took me out of the program. Since I was no longer fasting 6 days a week and getting sick on their supplements, I gained 80 pounds from February to May. I went from a cute size 6 to a size 20 prom dress. My weight exploded to 235lbs.

So, many of these behaviors followed me into adulthood. In front of people, I would eat all of the right things. I jumped on every band wagon of the latest and greatest diet plans. But on my own, I would binge. A crazy, vicious cycle. I guess, I always felt like I was trying to lose weight for someone else.

As a result of damage done to my metabolism due to the years of dieting and binging, I continued to gain weight at a rate of 40 pounds per year until I topped out somewhere around 375 lbs. I continued the same patterns and reinforced the behaviors that made every attempt at weight loss a total and utter failure. I still had not found a good enough "why?".

When I turned 26, all of that began to change. Even at my heaviest, I was relatively active and took aerobics classes and often walked on a treadmill or ran on an elliptical. My back began to strain under the excess weight and I began to have knee problems. Naturally concerned, I went to the chiropractor to have a routine consultation. When he was preparing the X-rays for review, I could tell there was legitimate concern on the doctor's face. He left the room and when he returned, he was carrying Kleenex. He pulled up the rolling stool, and took a seat by the exam table. He pursed his lips, looked me in the eye and said, "It isn't good. You have Stage 4 Degenerative Disk. You have to do something about your excess weight. You are 26. If you don't do something aggressive, your spinal column will collapse by the time you are 30 and you will be in a wheelchair. You will be lucky to live to the age of 40."

I don't remember the end of the appointment or the drive home, but I had most definitely discovered my "why?". That was the defining moment for me when weight loss evolved from a game I had played to a fight for my life. It became very real that my opportunity to change my life had a narrowing window. I took a hard look at myself. I was 26 years old. I looked at my life, and I had not begun to accomplish everything I wanted to in life, nor had I allow myself to live life to the fullest.

This moment, something awakened inside of me. The desire to overcome my weight, and create an extraordinary life filled every fiber of my being. I knew I had to change, and I have never looked back.

As you set out on your path of healthier living, once you know "what" you want, you MUST identify "why" you want it. This must be a powerful personal conviction that evokes a personal call to action. Your goal will either become your priority, or you will continue to lose at the diet games.

The "why" allows you to go past all previous superficial attempts. The fact that you failed before, no longer matters. The "why" gives roots to your goals anchoring them deep inside you. By connecting the goal to your inner self, you will have more strength, drive, and determination than you have ever experienced before during the process to reach your weight loss goals.

People ask me all the time, "how do you stay motivated?" Practice. I practice being motivated. I make a deliberate decision to be excited about the food I am eating, the portion control I have, or the fact that I am able to walk, run, and workout.

Enthusiasm to work out did not always come easily to me. In fact, I used to have severe gym anxiety. I would drive to the gym and sit in my car. Then, when I finally found the courage to go in, I would go inside, check in at the desk, walk a quick lap around the perimeter of the workout floor, then make a mad dash back to the safety of my car. Ladies and gentlemen, this was not at my highest weight, either. At the point, I had lost 100+ lbs. At my heaviest, I had TWO monthly paid gym memberships, but I would never make it through the door!

What changed was my mindset. I became grateful that I could walk, run, use the elliptical, or take a Zumba class. Every morning, we get a choice of how to tackle our day. Make a decision to be motivated. Practice happiness and excitement. You should live life as a celebration. If you have to....fake it until you make it. Motivation and positivity, just like success, are habits. Habits are learned behaviors. How you behave is a choice. Choose to be motivated and practice. Over time, your motivation will become contagious to others. Soon, people will start asking you how you stay motivated. Simply smile, and say, "Practice."

If you have never done so, take time to explore and understand "why" you really want to lose weight. Give yourself the opportunity to connect deeper to what drives you. Tap into your primal motivation.

Why do you want to lose weight? Has your health begun to suffer due to your added pounds? Perhaps, you dream of running a marathon? Are you a new mom, and you want to shed the baby weight and increase your energy? Do you want to rekindle the spark in your relationship? Maybe, you are tired of living for everyone else, and now is time to focus on you. Whatever it is that motivates you to achieve your goal, put it as the cornerstone of your journey and allow it to spur you to achievements that you had not realized were possible.

"Whatever you can do, or dream you can, begin it. Boldness

has genius, magic, and power in it."

Johann Wolfgang Von Goethe

ACTIVITY

Create a virtual vision board. Use a blank format PowerPoint slide, copy and paste images that represent your short, medium, and long term goals. Also, include images that illustrate "why" you want to meet these goals. Save a PPT copy on your desktop; so, as you achieve goals you can swap the images out with new goals. Save a PDF version and use this as the wallpaper for your desktop, laptop, tablet or Smart phone. If a picture is worth 1000 words, your vision board will tell volumes about how you want to grow your life.

See www.fromplussizetopinup.com_for more examples.

NOTES

_____

_____

_____

_____

_____

_____

_____

_____

_____

_____

_____

_____

_____

_____

_____

_____

_____

3

SO, NOW WHAT?

"Our goals can only be reached through a vehicle of a plan, in which we must fervently believe, and upon which we must vigorously act. There is no other route to success."

Stephen A. Brennan

The most critical effort to success is creating an action plan and sticking to it. To do that, here are the 4 steps I follow:

1) Break large goals into smaller, more manageable units.

2) Manage the units by time, inches, or pounds.

3) Reward yourself and celebrate the completion of each micro goal (non-food related rewards!!!)

4) Reevaluate goals after each achieved micro goal, repeat 1-3 until reaching the desired result.

We took time in the first two chapters to identify what we want and understand why we want it. The next phase is to determine how you will reach that goal. First, you must break down your BIG goals into smaller more manageable units. For example, if your goal is to lose 100 pounds, break it down into 10 x 10lbs weight loss sprints. Remember, success also depends on perspective. For some, the 10 pound sprint will be a motivator. For other, the scale may demotivate, so a better strategy would be monitoring success through inch loss or clothing size. Both are a fantastic jump start toward your personal goal...and technically both measure roughly the same success. Losing 10 pounds is roughly dropping a clothing size; however, it is the power of the perspective and method of viewing the journey that sparks motivation and will ultimately ignite success.

For me, I loved the 10 pound challenge. The process thrilled me to see the scale trickle down 9, 8, 6, 5, 3, 1....until I had lost another 10 pounds. I was competing mind against body; yet, now I realize it is actually conquer the mind and the body follows. Each time I reached a "0", I got excited to pass into a new set of numbers. The threshold of a new "ten" would motivate me to push harder and see the reduction in "decades" of weight loss as I viewed it. For the gamers out there, these became my weight loss "levels". Honestly, it did become a game to me and I enjoyed the satisfaction of conquering each level. If my weight loss started to slow, I learned to change my routine such as altering my diet, adding additional water, eventually cutting out soda, and increasing or changing my weekly activities. A change would always create a spike in my metabolism and my weight would continue to go down, down, down.

This strategy finally made weigh loss fun. I played detective to see what element in my diet or exercise regime needed change to generate a whole new round of weight loss. I learned to trick my body into shedding pounds. Remember, I knew I was in this for the long haul--my top weight was 375lbs and my first "BIG" goal was to reach 175lbs. But, by approaching the goal 10 pounds at a time, I was always successful. I created a habit of success. I trusted that I COULD lose weight. My journey became an intriguing puzzle to unlock rather than a self-proclaimed impossibility. Did my body change? Absolutely!!! However, the impact of my thoughts and attitude towards my body, healthy eating and the concept of weight loss -- that is where the true change occurred.

The process of weight loss became a journey of self-discovery and appreciation. I learned the natural rhythm of my body. The periodic fluctuations up and down -- those became a game, too. The focus of that game was to weigh less than the low of the previous month. If the low was lower, the monthly high would be lower, as well. I finally understood that the ebb and flow of a few pound was natural and healthy, so I no longer feared seeing the scale creep up a few pounds. This phenomenon was no longer a disaster, and so the negativity ceased.

I stopped comparing my weight loss to others. I continually lost about 3 to 7 pounds per month. At times, I would get discouraged when a beginning dieter would boast a 10-12 pound drop in their first week. Then, I realized, two weeks later, the beginner had run out of steam and had returned to the old eating habits. So, after two months, the boastful dieter would return to his/her original weight or higher, but I would be my consistent 6 to 14 pounds down the ticker. That is when I realized that I had declared success. I was winning the war.

So, how about you? The first week you were so good the pounds were jumping off the scale. How many of you have been the weekly warrior? Then, you perished in the flames of a birthday party binge? Wounded from your lack of self-control, you ditch the diet completely, do some comfort food damage, only to declare total defeat when the scale creeps back to its origin or perhaps carrying a bonus. I was this person for 28 years, until I said "STOP!"

Right now, I encourage you to "STOP" the madness. The awakening occurs when you realized that you went overboard in your food choices, but you must rid yourself of the "cheat" mentality. The mindset you must battle is guilt. So, you had a piece of birthday cake....that is no excuse to now ravage and binge the rest of the weekend. The mantra of "oh, well, I already blew it" is a lazy excuse to not accept control over one's food intake and through self-discipline out the window. Each additional splurge continues to stack up the guilt.....until you abandon the confines of the ideology of diet.

Well friends, it isn't the diet that is wrong nor that the body that doesn't respond to healthy eating. It is the mind that corrupts the efforts from the notion of the diet/binge cycle that creates a river of guilt. We build a food dam to hold back the raging waters of guilt. When the dam breaks, we abandon the diet and are left with feelings of failure and discontent, until the flood waters subside and we are willing to try again. Trust me, I am an expert on this cycle. I repeated it for over 20 years,

So, how do you defeat that cycle?

1) Control your food intake. If that breaks down, and you indulge

2) Control your emotions. Do not allow temporary disappointment in your food choices spiral you out of control.

3) Control your journey and jump immediately back on your food and exercise plan.

Guess what? A *minor* slip can actually boost your metabolism and weigh loss. Just know that jumping back on track will minimize the effects of the indiscretion and could promote additional fat loss, especially if it was an out of the norm indulgence. Remember, what you do 95% of the time is what will create success. So, STOP beating yourself up over the 5%. But keep it in perspective...if the 5% creeps into a higher percentage of your routine, you are slipping back into old habits. Make the adjustments necessary to refocus and get back on track, but don't give in to guilt. The bad habit that has robbed you of success for far too long. Be proud of your new behaviors of self-reflection and self-evaluation.

Finally, you MUST reward yourself. We are conditioned to praise good behaviors. We praise our spouses, children, co-workers, and even the dog on a job well done. Yet, do we intentionally praise ourselves? When was the last time you truly did something nice for yourself? I'm not talking about a splurge in a moment of weakness, or that sale that you could not pass up....or even getting your hair or nails done or car detailed. You should do that because it feels good to look your best. I am talking about placing time and attention on yourself for the explicit purpose to celebrate something that you accomplished.

"We cannot grow when we are in shame, and we can't use shame to change ourselves or others."

Brené Brown

ACTIVITY

Positive self-talk is more powerful than you can imagine.

Search YouTube go to guided meditation or personal

affirmations. Find one that connects to you

Start every morning with an hour of meditation and positive

affirmations for 30 days. Play the video or mp3 on the

background of your phone or computer, even with

earphones, and go about your morning, every morning.

After 30 days, evaluate and reflect on how you evolved

personally, professionally, and in relationships.

Dare to make a difference. Here is to a:

happier, healthier, more positive and prosperous life!

NOTES

_____

_____

_____

_____

_____

_____

_____

_____

_____

_____

_____

_____

_____

_____

_____

_____

4

EYES ON THE PRIZE

"The only people capable of handling success are those who have learned to handle failures without taking their eyes off the prize."

Orrin Woodward

Make it BIG. Make it important. Make it intentional.

For every micro-goal achieved. Reward yourself. Make sure it is a reward that will keep you focused day by day until you cash it in. Don't make it a food reward. That will create confusion in the mind toward the new health eating. Instead, it would reinforce the diet = punishment, favorite treat = reward cycle that you must break for long term, continued success. Finally, make it something really cool and really meaningful to you. As soon as you celebrate you, step forward into the path toward the next micro-goal and set a new exciting reward. Success after success, motivation will be abundant.

I started my weight loss journey in the spring of 2008. I had committed to myself that I would begin my journey to free myself from the grasp of the fat lady holding my life hostage. I knew that the journey would be long. I knew I had never succeeded before....but I knew, as a matter of life, or death, I HAD to succeed this time. I knew that I needed to stay motivated. (Odd that life or death isn't enough of a motivator. Sadly, how many diabetics or people with heart disease refuse to follow the recommended health plan from their physicians? These choices can also mean a more immediate life or death scenarios, and still old habits die hard. It is human nature to find success when there is excitement surrounding the journey. Dietary restrictions mandated by a physician are not sexy or fun. Initially the scare tactic can lead people to temporary changes, but those even are usually short lived. Self-motivation is the key to long term pursuit of a goal. Rewards help keep motivation growing throughout the process.

I needed a reward system. I used to use smaller clothing sizes to motivate my weight loss, but I was a long way from a size 6. I had practiced this method for over a decade and had a bedroom closet full of smaller sizes to "work my way into". At this time in my life, my skinny jeans were no match for temptation....a cup cake would win every time. I realized that this type of goal setting was not effective for me. I needed something HUGE to keep me on track. Help me resist the urge to cheat and important enough that it would stay in the back of my mind to help me push through the cake in the breakroom type of days.

I began to exchange my appetite for food for an appetite for life. I realized my weight and my perception had deprived me of so many of life's experiences. For example, when I was 21, I took a summer Biology course in Costa Rica. An amazing trip with amazing people. We hiked volcanoes, rode horses through cloud forests and body surfed with baby black fin sharks. Some would say that even at 300 pounds, I knew how to get the most out of life. The highlight of the trip was zip lining through the canopy. We stood in line getting fit with our harness and our gear. As the line dwindled and it was my time to be fit, I held my breath. The attendant tugged, pulled and twisted the harness; then, he turned to my professor Paulo and had a side-bar conversation. With compassion, Paulo pulled me aside and tenderly explained that they did not have a harness big enough to allow me to participate. Even if they could get the harness to close, it would not hold. Wounded, I choked back big tears, embarrassed that I was to be left behind, but more humiliated that my peers watched the event and silently understood that it was because I was too fat. I knew at that moment, one day I would conquer the weight and remove all limitations it had placed on my life. And, so I have.

The struggle with food addiction is a highly emotional one. So, if the reward has an emotional element to it, the impact of the reward on the level of motivation will skyrocket. As I began to lose weight, I began to schedule activities that I spent years avoiding. I used these events as motivators to nudge me ever further on my journey. Simple formula. Anything, everything I wanted to do. I began to do. Travel, dancing, concerts, amusement parks, events. I created a cycle of success, the by product was fun --but the true reward was a healthier, happier me.

Set your rewards. Make them significant to you. Do what you need to do to stay motivated. Apologize to no one for your reward choices....no matter how crazy or extreme it may be--the purpose is to keep YOU motivated. Achieve your goals and reap your rewards. This process is good for any success cycle and can be applied to all areas of life. The more you make the micro-goal/reward cycle work for you, success will be more and more predominant in your life. Visit my website and join the community. See how others stay motivated, share strategies, and inspire others. You will empower others because you choose to empower yourself. www.melissawritesstuff.com/community

"A strong mind focuses not on its obstacle, but on the reward that lies at the end of it."

Edmond Mbiaka

ACTIVITY

Book your first reward activity to correspond with the deadline of your first micro-goal.

As you cash in each reward by achieving the goal, schedule the next reward. Variety is the spice of life. Change it up, make each reward exciting and different. Trade in your appetite for food with an appetite for life.

Make it BIG. Make it important.

Make it intentional.

NOTES

_____

_____

_____

_____

_____

_____

_____

_____

_____

_____

_____

_____

_____

_____

_____

5

SOCIAL YIN/YANG

"Don't let the opinions of the average man sway you. Dream, and he thinks you're crazy. Succeed, and he thinks you're lucky. Pay no attention. He simply doesn't understand."

Robert G Allen

As you start to make positive changes in your life, you may encounter a mixture of positive and negative reactions from your friends, relatives, and peers. Everyone will have an opinion and perception as your body begins to morph to a fitter, sleeker silhouette. As if it is not challenging enough to overcome self-sabotage, to eliminate negative influences from outside sources can be a challenge as you begin to move beyond the comfort zone of the way you have always done things. You must train yourself to identify these mindset terrorists, understand their motives; then, build your strategy to overcome the situation and find justice for yourself.

The naysayer:

This individual may begin negative remarks to you once he/she notices a change in your behavior as well as your physical transformation. This individual usually feels stuck in a rut and does not see/feel success in his/her own life. Therefore, there is no way this person can visualize someone else succeeding. My most challenging naysayer came in the form of my physician. He told me that "due to the extreme nature of my obesity and the severe damage I had done to my metabolism, the best I could hope for was to reach a goal weight of 225 lbs." I felt my lips purse, eyes water, and throat tighten to choke back my sobbing. I wanted to get to 175 lbs. My doctor had just told me that it was an impossibility. Instead of accepting his prediction for my fate, I used my rage to fuel my fire. How dare he tell me that I won't reach my goal. Part of my motivation was simple to prove my doctor wrong. Perhaps that was his goal, I will never be sure; however, I met his goal for me of 225 lbs., continued on to my goal of 175 lbs. Then, I reevaluated and realized, I was not finished. Today, I weigh 140 lbs. This is 85 lbs. less than what the doctor said was even possible. Do not let anyone determine your fate. It is entirely up to you to create the life you want. I am here to remind you that the impossible is indeed possible, and your potential is so much more than you realized when you began. The naysayer comes in several forms. The individuals who don't believe you will success. Some will say it while other show their attitude toward your success. The naysayer may say that your goals are not possible. This person may even downplay your success by calling you "lucky" or justifying his/her own failures. Do not let this person poison your positivity. Success is your choice, not theirs.

The "emotional crutch":

This individual is afraid of change. He/she is a lifetime member of the "yo-yo" diet society. He/she thrives on group failure. This may be the person that organizes group or office weight loss challenges, but his/her favorite topic is "weigh in" day and "how much so and so has cheated this week". This is usually the person who thrives on self-sabotage and when you are showing results, will be the first to tempt you to cheat since "you are doing so well....you can allow yourself to eat

_____(fill in the blank with whatever food he/she is offering at that moment)." Hold your ground, and keep your focus. Once you are finished reading, you should offer to let him/her to borrow this book.

The "extremist/health nut":

This individual is up to date on all the latest fitness trends. He/she may view your efforts as haphazard and half-way.

He/she will always have the "best" advice, as they believe everyone should train and eat like Mr. Olympia. Do not let this individual discourage you because "you aren't there, yet" or you don't assume such an extreme way of life. Small changes getting started add to the results lasting for a lifetime. If you decide to train for fitness competitions and such, you have the power to do so. Go for it! If not, don't let extremists shake your confidence about the positive changes and efforts you are making in your own lifestyle. Also, don't let the "experts" distract you with method after method and trying one approach after another. A diet, workout routine or combo needs a minimum of 90 days to get maximum results, at that point it will be time to switch it up to keep the body active and continue to boost fat loss.

The "coach":

This individual is also on a weight loss journey. He/she will find interest in yours, as well. This person will check in often and discuss and compare weight loss results. This individual has

great intentions to motivate you. Just remember, everyone

loses weight at a different pace. Depending on the focus of the

conversation, be careful that the focus does not solely rely on

pounds/inches lost. Especially if one of you is losing faster than

the other, it can cause some unhealthy competition and

insecurity. Instead, focus on the process. Discuss the new

healthy recipe you tried or the new class at the gym you like.

Positive support can be highly motivating.

The "mother hen":

Another individual with good intentions is the "mother hen".

This individual, male or female finds an irresistible urge to feed

people.... food and hospitality are the "mother hen's" love

language. Once, the "mother hen" notices your progress, it will

become his/her mission to make sure nothing is wrong and you

are eating healthy. Honesty is the best approach with the

"mother hen". Explain that you are working towards better health and ensure them that you are eating a well-balanced, nutritious diet. They may resist for a while and keep offering large portions or snacks for a while. They will finally accept your transformation.

The "social butterfly":

This individual is a great deal of fun. He/she does not intend on increasing your struggle, but let's face it...99% of social activities revolve around food or drinks. Change the pace and make suggestions of non-food related get-togethers. If food is on the agenda; then, prep yourself ahead of time. Look online at the menu and decide the best choices to keep you on track. On the day of the meet up, make sure to drink plenty of water and don't skip any meals. If you go to dinner hungry, appetite might take over and you may abandon the original plan for ordering. Instead, stick to the game plan. The more successful outings you have staying on track, the more confident and enthused you will stay about your new healthier habits. Your transformation is about living life to the fullest extent, never missing a moment, and letting your life shine. You do not have to avoid social activities to avoid temptation. Focus on the fun, not the food. Who knows? You might be the social butterfly in your group. Leave the cocoon and show your true colors.

The "late night snacker":

There is always *THAT* friend, or in my case husband, that wants to grab a late night snack. Don't feel obligated to participate in the late night binge. Drink a glass of water when you arrive. Evaluate your hunger level. Are you really hungry, or are you trying to fill the emotional delusion of normalcy by ordering a full meal? If you are truly hungry, order a soup, salad, or small portion of a side item that would satisfy your immediate craving. If you are not hungry, don't feel guilty about not ordering. Get a coffee or a hot tea to provide as a comfortable

70

conversation companion, but do not mindlessly eat before bedtime. It is a waste of money and unnecessary consumption. If you feel guilty, leave the server the tip of the amount of the food you would have purchased. There, you will show generosity and you look out for the best interest of your body.

The "Cheerleader": This individual has positive energy and is highly supportive. This person is always there to offer a smile and an encouraging word. He/she is a gem in anyone's life. However, do not let the cheerleader distract you from your goal. The cheerleader in your life loves you as you are and sees you through rose colored glasses. So, he/she may give you so many compliments about your success that it may influence compromise. You may start justifying cheat days and splurges because you have "come so far." Do not fall into that trap. Those behaviors throw you back to the habit of rewarding with food. So, embrace the cheerleader in your life and bask in the positivity, but reject complacency. Recognize the role the cheerleader plays in your life, but keep an optimistic realism to keep your goals in check. Remember, the journey is by you and for you to enhance your health, happiness, and lifestyle.

There will be other characters and situations that will cross your pathway on your journey to the best you. These examples are a guide to start looking at each person or situation and analyze the relationship to you, your health, and your happiness. If someone is being negative to you, nine times out of ten, it is a reflection of the person and the attitude he/she has chosen to express that day, week, or period of time. Therefore, don't take it personally and don't get insulted. The person's reaction to you reflects more about how they feel about him/herself. So, do not waste an ounce of energy letting him/her affect the attitude with which you have chosen to embrace the world. Finally, do not fear that the changes you are making to become healthier will destroy your social life or limit the experiences you can have. On the contrary, be bold, be fierce, plan ahead, choose better, design the life you want to live and live it abundantly. Life becomes so liberating when you realize that happiness is your choice. So, what are you waiting for? Live happy.

"Today I am in control because I want to be. I have my fingers on the switch, but have lived a lifetime ignoring the control I have over my own world. Today is different."

A.S. King, *Please Ignore Vera Dietz*

ACTIVITY

As you begin to reflect on the people in your life and how they impact and influence your mindset. Go a step further. Discover who you are for other people. Make it a practice to be the positive breath of fresh air in a world full of negativity. Be the Success Enthusiast, encourage and hold friends accountable to what they say the wish to accomplish. Be candid. If someone is stuck in a diet/health Ferris wheel. Openly say, listen, I care about you, and I know you can succeed in reaching your goals. When you are truly ready to be/do _____, nothing will stop your success. It all goes back to "how badly do you want it."

He/she may be taken back or mad at first, but they will respect that you called his/her bluff. Encourage your friends to have this type of candor with you, as well. Create an accountability circle and watch mountains move.

NOTES

6

SHAMPOO, RINSE, AND REPEAT

"The less routine, the more life."

Amos Bronson Alcott

Everyone knows the definition of insanity; why do we stick to the status quo and expect a revolution?

Lessons learned from a shampoo bottle: I have fine, blonde hair. I struggle with finding the perfect Shampoo and Conditioner that will give me enough moisture to make my hair soft and is not so heavy that it will weigh it down. I switch from brand to brand looking for the holy grail of hair products. Recently, I read an article that suggests that fine haired individuals should condition first for a few minutes, then shampoo. It works perfectly every time.

I have read the directions on thousands of Shampoo and Conditioner bottles, and followed standard industry practice for over 30 years. The products were never the issue; the routine was the problem. With the most insignificant change, I now have salon perfect beach waves. Sometimes it takes the smallest disruption of order to obtain the most significant results.

The same goes with diet and exercise. You do not have to do a complete overhaul of lifestyle to create the results you want in your life. But, you must start with something and create a pattern of consistency.

Growing up in Texas, there are two preferred beverages – Sweet Tea and Dr. Pepper. Please, ask any Texan, you will get the same response. In high school, I drank a 6 pack of Dr. Pepper every day. At that time in my life, I did not like the "taste" of water, and stuck to my daily regimen of 72 oz. of soda per day. If I was drinking Sweet Tea, I easily consumed half a gallon. With this detail alone, I was not detoxing the body by drinking proper fluids. The caffeine contributed to water retention due to chronic dehydration. Through liquids alone, I was consuming 1000 additional unnecessary calories every day. In a year, that is 365,000 calories or approximately 104 pounds of extra weight. If I had made this single change, this book may never have been written.

So think about it. If you are currently overweight, something in your routine isn't working to your advantage. Start implementing the direct, obvious changes you can do. For example, trade your beverage consumption to drinking water. If that seems to bland for your pallet, add essential oils or fruit to create "spa water" with additional health benefits. Hey, sometimes you have to get creative to get motivated. Monitor your results, when the improvements start to slow down, you know it is time to implement a new change of habit. Tackle them one at a time, and make them stick. Slow and steady will win the race, as they are no longer a diet, but a lifestyle. Wash, Rinse, and Repeat this cycle until you achieve your optimum health goals.

Another reason for blah results is boredom! If cheating on a diet or focus on "forbidden fruit" is one of your toughest daily struggles, you are probably bored with your routine. Your mind needs stimulation, and the quickest, instant gratification is through food. Start feeding your mind with all the colors of life.

The mind can be enriched through color, fragrance, art, nature, literature, music, dance, theatre, film and culture. How often do you incorporate these activity into your life? You don't have to be a billionaire to experience the finer things in life. Simply look around you and see what your city has to offer. I live in Southern California, so I make sure that a week does not go by that we don't attend an event, explore a new park or garden, go to a museum, and walk daily along the shoreline. Activities such as these break the routine. They give a higher value to my life quality and I have a greater sense of balance in my life.

It is exhilarating to break the 4th wall of your life and experience an activity out of the norm to acknowledge all of the realities that coexist in the world. For me, I can get lost in the thoughts and the ponderings of my own mind for hours. A luxury I missed for so many years as I was enslaved to food.

Life is busy. There are ample schedules and responsibilities, but how much life are you missing or are you letting pass by you, because you are too busy to notice or consumed with addictions to care? These life experiences are great to use as motivators for your reward system, but more that you are creating a multi-sensory lifestyle that will breathe new life into all of your day to day activities.

We get one clean shot at life on this planet. I determined very early that I would not dedicate my life to a grey cubical experiencing what I know about the world from Google, Wikipedia, and social media. That was not enough for me. I created a job that gave me the freedom and flexibility. Since I am always on my own schedule, I can include these sensory indulgences whenever something pops up that I want to see or do. In essence, to live a life filled with success find balance with diet, work, lifestyle and finally fitness.

For me, fitness was the biggest challenge to overcome. The leftover insecurities of my formal self would often drip into my thoughts and make me believe that I don't belong at the gym, or that everyone is staring at me while I exercise. Let me set the record straight, no one is judging you at the gym. It is a narcissistic haven where everyone is wrapped up in their own image and how they are being perceived. If you

84

don't have time to spend additional time on you, why would a stranger devote their time and energy to devote to perceiving you. Just saying!

Again, with fitness, you do not have to start at the gym, but start somewhere. I love to walk, and with the luxury of living in a beach city, my favorite stroll is to a lighthouse. It is 45 minute to an hour, and I know I have hit my activity goal for that day. If I want to mix it up, I add activities throughout the week, but in addition to walking, not instead of it.

This may take some creativity and strategy on your part, but make activity an integral part of your day. Have gratitude for the ability to use your body, run, play dive, and skip. To some, mobility would be a luxury; so who are we not to enjoy the freedom to move? One of my favorite quotes is "he that does not read good books is no different than one who cannot read them." Think about it, neither is using the mind to read. The same goes for the body. If you do not use your body, you are no different than someone who cannot use his/her body. Remember, mobility is not forever, what if one day, all of that changes through an accident, illness, or injury. Would you have regrets? Did you push your limits and life physically to your greatest capacity? Typically, only one out of ten will answer "yes."

So what are you waiting for? Make life delicious.

A mind that is stretched by a new experience can never go back to its old dimensions.

Oliver Wendell Holmes, Jr.

ACTIVITY

Break the monotony! Try one new recipe, activity, and
workout every week for the next 6 weeks. During that
timeframe, you will have broadened your horizon to 18 new
experiences. The ones you like, add them to your current
favorites. The ones you don't. Move on, but at least you tried
something new!

NOTES

_____

_____

_____

_____

_____

_____

_____

_____

_____

_____

_____

_____

_____

_____

_____

_____

7

IS THAT ALL YOU'RE WORTH?

"We can reverse years of damage to our bodies by deciding to raise our standards for ourselves, then living differently. Old wounds heal, injuries repair, and the whole system improves with just a few changes in what we put into our bodies and how we move them."

Anonymous

If you reflect back toward the beginning of the book, I outlined my diagnosis of Stage 4 Degenerative Disk Disease. Remember, if I did not do something (and I did), my spinal column was going to buckle under my tremendous weight.

So, what happens when 4 years pass, 176 pounds have been dropped (I wanted to wait until I dropped under the 200 pound mark, known to many obesity advocacy groups as onederland)? Afraid of what I would hear, and to know the extent damage my years of bodily abuse, I finally scheduled a checkup with a Chiropractor. I went in for the full workup. This time; however, it was me who was awkward and nervous. The doctor came in all smiles ready to discuss my treatment. I braced myself for the worst. "Well, miss Glossup, there is some crowding and stress in the upper neck and some misalignment in the lower lumbar. Treatment will be effective in as few as 6 visits."

"What about the degeneration? How bad is it?" I asked.

"Degeneration? There is no evidence of degeneration, the discs are normally spaced with a bit of stress in the neck and lower back, nothing to be too concerned about."

Like a Catholic in confession, I shared the story of my last visit, informed him of my weight loss journey. He showed me the X-Rays and reassured me… my back had made a full recovery. Losing the weight allowed the pressure on the discs to release, and there was no indication of degeneration.

With gratitude, I walked to my car, a bit overwhelmed by the news I had received. The human body has an amazing capacity for healing! At that moment, I realized it is never too late to revamp a situation in your life; and with that thought, all the fear subsided from my body. I knew the only limitations in this life are the ones that you allow to take hold and control you. No, no. Not me. Not anymore. Not in this lifetime!

That was my Independence Day. I'm not going to tell you every day has been peaches and positivity, because it hasn't. Don't get me wrong. Life is an incredible, amazing journey. People assume that weight loss was my main focus. Yes, changing my lifestyle became a part of who I am. However, during my physical downsizing, moved from Texas to California, juggled 3 jobs, wrote 4 US Patent application, co-founded a corporation and developed new, innovative wearable technology. So, when someone tells me that he/she is too busy to eat well or workout, I have little sympathy for their apathy. Like Parkinson's law suggests, "work expands so as to fill the **time** available for its completion". So, if someone really wants to accomplish a goal, it will become a priority and time will be allotted for its completion.

I am also not going to tell you that I was the perfect epitome of diet and exercise at every moment over the past few years; but remember, what matters is what you do 95% of the time. After all, you have to live life. The problem lurks when you allow past habits to creep in and you look for reasons to increase 5% to, say, 25%. At that point, you should take a moment to reevaluate and jump back on track, or have a few close friends that you trust to hold you accountable.

One of my most insightful reality checks came to me through my husband. I had more than exceeded my share of splurges for the week. I was caught between the demands of running a startup technology company and teaching full time. I was walking and whining to my husband when I made the declaration, " I am having a rough day, I DESERVE a Frappuccino!"

He turned, disgusted, looked at me and said, "That's all you're worth?"

Silence. As I thought about what he said, I envisioned where I began my journey. I had spent so much time nurturing obesity but ignoring my emotions. Like a movie reel, all of my failures and accomplishments flashed across my mind. Reflecting on my life and how far I had come, he was right. I had given food the power to substitute my own feelings of self-worth. There was an is no food or substance that should take priority over my health and well-being. No splurge or snack should act as a bandage to my emotional health. For far too long, I had found comfort in food. That day, my relationship changed with the way I allowed my mind to relate to food. I realized that I need to address and acknowledge my emotions, then deal with it.

Luckily, though the years it took to erase the excess fat from my form, I had learned to become self-reflective. Through evaluation, I began to understand what was good for my body, why I did not lose weight this week, or how to jumpstart my metabolism out of a lull.

Self-reflection has been the key to my success. Now, the process of being self-reflective moved beyond the physiology of weight reduction, but to really understand "why?" I had this relationship with food. I have a greater understanding of who I am and why I am. An individual should ideally be a balance of mind, body, and spirit. The mind I conquered at a young age through education. Body wise, at this time, I had spent 4 years restoring balance. The last unknown frontier was my emotions. Truly, it was like meeting myself for the first time. In a way it is funny, I am an incredible friend, but I had never given myself the time of day. As I began addressing my emotions, cravings stopped. I had more control, and found it easy to lose weight.

Here is the secret sauce to my success: the most important relationship you will ever have is with yourself.

This epiphany took 7 years of revelation. Within the relationship with the self, three elements must be addressed:

1) Self-love – how you treat yourself.

2) Self-respect – how you take care of your physical needs.

3) Self efficacy – what you believe you can do.

If individuals focus to develop these three elements, weight and obesity would be a non-issue, because the behaviors that lead to obesity would not be tolerated by someone who creates harmony within.

Make yourself a priority. Stop compromising. No excuses.

"You yourself, as much as anybody in the entire universe, deserve your love and affection"

Gautama Buddha

ACTIVITY

What about you? How is your weight effecting your life? What impact in your life would you experience if you lost the extra weight? What do you have to lose? For every aspect in your life that losing weight will improve, create a tree diagram that shows all of the life possibilities that can manifest to enrich your life. Ex:

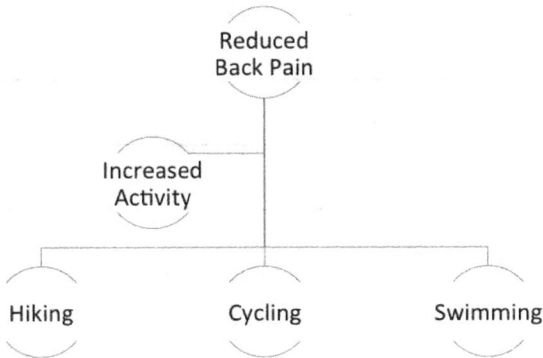

NOTES

8
START AN EVOLUTION

"Every single cell in the human body replaces itself over a period of seven years. That means there's not even the smallest part of you now that was part of you seven years ago."

Steven Hall

Seven years ago, I took the first steps towards changing my life. Today, I stand on the other end of that pathway, healthy, thin, successful, and more alive than I have ever been. I am completely regenerated, renewed, and reinvented.

In life, there is either growth or decay, but nothing remains the same. As you choose what to do with the insights found in this book, I hope you find encouragement and inspiration in your journey.

As I writing this book, I want to highlight that in order to create an optimal life, you must develop a healthy self-respect. You cannot lose an addiction or break a bad habit by creating a sole focus on the problem. However, the SOLUTION is you. If you divert the wasted negative energy from the yo-yo dieting cycle, and empower yourself to enrich your mind, engage your body, and elevate your spirit, the physical maladies of obesity will ultimately fade away. The more you release yourself from the traditional stresses of dieting, you will gain the freedom to create the life you want.

ACTIVITY

Write an encouraging letter to yourself dated 7 years forward. Describe the life you want: health, house, family, career, etc. For example, "You selected a beautiful 4 bedroom beachfront cottage to raise your family." For additional content, take the notes you kept while reading the book, and create the story of your what and why. Tell yourself how proud you are that you took the steps to change your life. You understand the courage and dedication it takes to change your mindset and redirect your life Include and detail any vision you wish to see in your future self. Place the letter in a sealed envelope and date it to be opened on the same date 7 years from now. keep the letter in a cabinet or a safe hidden drawer. Seeing the letter from time to time will be a surprising motivator. Finally, when the date arrives to read the letter, you will connect to your former self and appreciate the change you have created. This is for your eyes only. Give yourself the attention you deserve.

7 KEY SRATEGIES

Through my experiences, there are 7 Key Strategies for permanent weight loss success.

7. Take ACTION – Get started fresh each day. One day at a time and each day unto itself. Never, never give up.

6. Set SMART GOALS.

Specific, Measurable, Attainable, Relevant, Timely

5. REWARD milestones throughout your journey.

4. SELF-REFLECTION to drive results.

3. POSSITIVE AFFIRMATIONS to develop positive self-talk and empower the voice within.

2. GRATITUDE magnify your life to abundance.

1. Increase your SELF-WORTH

Promise Yourself

To be so strong that nothing
can disturb your peace of mind.
To talk health, happiness, and prosperity
to every person you meet.

To make all your friends feel
that there is something in them
To look at the sunny side of everything
and make your optimism come true.

To think only the best, to work only for the best,
and to expect only the best.
To be just as enthusiastic about the success of others
as you are about your own.

To forget the mistakes of the past
and press on to the greater achievements of the
future.
To wear a cheerful countenance at all times
and give every living creature you meet a smile.

To think well of yourself and to proclaim this fact to
the world,
not in loud words but great deeds.
To live in faith that the whole world is on your side
so long as you are true to the best that is in you.

Christian D. Larson

NOTES

_____

_____

_____

_____

_____

_____

_____

_____

_____

_____

_____

_____

_____

_____

_____

_____

MELISSA MICHELLE GLOSSUP MA, MED

BONUS

INTERVIEW

TIPS & TRICKS

HELPFUL LINKS

INTERVIEW

Karen Langston, Certified Holistic Nutritionist creator of the Nutrition Advisor and Healthy Gut Advisor Program

1) Is the obesity epidemic worsening in the US? What do you believe the main cause(s) of this is/are?

The obesity epidemic globally affects 2.1 billion people worldwide. Obesity in the US and those who are overweight jumped to 27.5% for adults and 47.1% for children from 1980 to 2013 according to Institute for Health Metrics and Evaluation at the University of Washington. http://www.wsj.com/articles/nearly-30-of-world-population-is-overweight-1401365395   And, a shocking 42 million children under the age of 5 were overweight or obese in 2013. http://www.who.int/mediacentre/factsheets/fs311/en/

According to the McKinsey Global Institute global obesity epidemic is costing the world economy $2 trillion a year in health-care costs. http://www.mckinsey.com/insights/economic_studies/how_the_world_could_better_fight_obesity

The sad part about these statistics are the fact that obesity is a preventable condition.

Although the experts relate the problem of obesity to diet and lack of exercise, a ton of research also indicates the lack of the right gut microbiota that can affect metabolism. More than this, I believe the obesity epidemic is the lack of properly educating ourselves and acting upon the results to create change. Awareness is the key to action. And action creates lifesaving positive effects.

We are bombarded with a plethora of convenient packaged foods toting low calorie, no fat, low fat, sugar free, easy low calorie snack packs, drive-thrus with special low calorie menus. We drink skinny lattes, sugar free soft drinks all the while packing on the pounds. Why? Because we have become a nation that believes in the clever claims food companies put on their packages at face value; and yet, our waistlines continue to expand. It is like we are being set up for failure.

These are the main causes and, we know them quite well. What needs to change is our response to the information. We need to take action. We need to read third party information like books on health and nutrition knowing the author does not have a vested interest in the food industry. These books will give you the truth about how the ingredients and types of foods are negatively impacting your health.

We need to start exercising. It is an inexpensive way to stay healthy; all you need is 30 minutes a day and a pair of shoes. We need to start eating whole foods that do not contain ingredients that were concocted in a chemistry lab. We need to start now.

2) Childhood obesity is a rising concern, what should parents do for the nutrition of their children to help curb this phenomenon?

In order to take control of childhood obesity, parents need to lead by example. You can't expect a child to eat broccoli if the parent is eating French fries. Children are sponges and they learn by example. Start educating yourself by reading nutrition books, take a cooking class; better yet, take a cooking class with your child.

Learn to read the label for ingredients instead of calories. Calories do not represent what is in the package; calories are NOT created equal. Find nutritionists that do not have a vested interest in the fast food or refined food industry that can help in getting your family healthy. Look for a health practitioner, health coach or nutritionist that recommends whole foods over packaged foods. Parents need to learn how to really fill their children with quality nutrition. For example frozen chicken fingers may look like a low calorie option along with, low sodium and fat free; however, what is the nutrient deficit? If you remove the marketing hype "low sodium, fat free, under 10 calories" what is truly left? This is where you need to move beyond the calorie label and look at what is really in the package; the ingredient list is where to start. If the ingredient list contains words that you cannot pronounce and you do not know what it is; how do you think your body is going to utilize it?

If the label can't tell you what vitamins and minerals along with antioxidants are in the package, why would you want to eat it? For example organic "pasture raised" chicken that you cut up yourself and bread with ground almond flour will contain naturally occurring omega 3 fatty acids, calcium, magnesium, iron, vitamin B6 and a good source of protein. Whereas a typical frozen package of chicken fingers will contain genetically modified fed chicken with synthetic fortified government regulated vitamins along with bleached genetically modified wheat flour and other additives, preservatives and stabilizers. Which do you think will give you a better nutritional bang for your buck?

Emulsifiers are added to most processed foods to extend shelf life as well as make things creamier and give that satisfying full fat feel in the mouth. Most packaged foods will contain some form of an emulsifier especially creamy items like pudding, ice cream and even yogurt. Studies on mice indicate the chemicals that make up emulsifiers can alter gut bacteria (our microbiota) potentially causing significant weight gain leading to metabolic syndrome and even inflammatory bowel dissease.
http://dailysciencejournal.com/emulsifiers-in-processed-foods-may-cause-obesity-and-ibd/21429/
The ingredients in most packaged foods in fast food and restaurant food contain additional ingredients that can lead to not only obesity but other illness and even cancer. Most ingredients found in our processed foods have not been properly tested and studied.

3) What are 5 simple changes someone can make to move toward healthier nutrition and trim the waistline?

A. Exercise. I know most families lead busy lives; however, scheduling movement for 30 minutes a day is a must. For some families, going for a walk after dinner is all it takes. It is also a great way to bond spending quality time together. It also connects you with nature rebalancing mind, body and spirit. If this is not an option, enroll kids in some form of an activity that gets them moving at least one hour, 3 times a week. This will increase good mood and self-esteem. And, make sure parents are leading by example and are also creating movement or exercising.

B. We need to be getting at least 6-8 hours of sleep a night. Children need on average 8-10 hours of sleep. Sleep affects everything in the body including hormones and emotional balance. This directly impacts food choices. Sleep disruption in the body's circadian rhythm can lead to obesity. The lack of proper sleep triggers adrenal glands to produce cortisol. Elevated cortisol boosts insulin levels. Insulin is our response to sugar in the body and how the body deals with it.

Insulin is a hormone made by the pancreas that takes the sugar from your carbohydrates (like rice, pasta, flour products and even brown rice and other grains), breaks them down into simple sugars know as glucose. Glucose is used to create energy, feed your brain as well store energy for future use (in the form of fat). Insulin plays a major role in regulating carbohydrate and fat metabolism.

High levels of cortisol over time alters energy metabolism. When insulin and cortisol are constantly "running" this leads to increased cravings for carbohydrates, caffeine and sugar. Too much circulating sugar leads to fat storage. All this from not getting adequate sleep leads to increased cravings and increased fat storage especially, in the abdominal area and thighs.

C. Learn how to make food and freeze. This sounds so daunting, but it so rewarding. When I was a single mother, working full time and going to school, as well as, keeping up with my daughter's demanding skating lessons and competitions, fast food seemed convenient. Knowing the detriment of these types of foods, I just could not do that to my child or myself. Here is what I did to keep up the demands of a busy life and still eat nutritiously.

When I made dinner I would make extra for the next day or to freeze for another day. I would put the food into a glass container that could go from the freezer to fridge to thaw to the oven or into a pot on the stove to be reheated.

I also had a crockpot. The night before I would prepare the meal in the crockpot (this usually took about 10 minutes of my time). The next morning I would take the crockpot out of the fridge, and pop it into the sleeve, turn it on for the longest setting and would have a hot home cooked meal when we got home. The extras would become lunch or dinner the next evening or I would freeze into single glass containers for another night.

I also had an automated rice cooker and vegetable steamer with timers. Why would you want to do this? You eliminate all of the ingredients that could be contributing weight gain and cut down on your drive-thru options!

D. Take one vegetable you do not normally eat and turn it into a family project. Have one child of the appropriate age research the food item and give a mini presentation. Have another child research a recipe either in print or watch on YouTube. YouTube is really handy for showing you step-by-step how to make a recipe. As a family go grocery shopping for the ingredients to make the recipe. Once there is involvement there is more excitement and better chance of actually liking the food item and making it a part of a healthier lifestyle. And, as your "produce vocabulary" increases the less reliance on processed refined foods that are contributing to unhealthy waist lines.

E. Supplementation is a must! I know some of the medical profession and even dietician's feel that if you eat right you can get your nutrients from the food you eat. I beg to differ. We can clearly see by our expanding waist lines and the raise in inflammatory conditions such as diabetes, cardiovascular disease and inflammatory bowel disease we are confused about eating properly.

The SAD diet (Standard American Diet) contains genetically modified foods, grown in pesticide laden nutrient deficient soil, that have been manipulated, and contain synthetic nutrients and chemical concoctions to keep us coming back for more that are processed with fillers and extracts devoid of the vitamins, minerals and antioxidants we need on a daily bases.

We need to get back to organic farming practices and eat organic foods. A Newcastle University study on organic versus conventional crops found that there are substantially higher levels of antioxidants in fruits, vegetables, and grains, with some having as much as 60 percent higher concentrations of antioxidant compounds than conventional crops.http://www.ncbi.nlm.nih.gov/pubmed/24968103

Another study found that organic crops contained significantly more vitamin C, iron, magnesium, phosphorus and better essential amino acid content in comparison to their conventional grown crops. http://ucanr.edu/datastoreFiles/608-794.pdf

So, my point here is unless you are eating 100% organic produce, grains, grass fed, pasture raised meat and poultry, drink clean quality water and have no stress you need to supplement.

The basic foundation is fiber, probiotics, a good liver support, fish oil and a good quality multi/mineral complex. Fiber bulks up the colon, wraps around toxins and excess estrogens and takes them out of our body. Toxins and excess estrogens including xenoestrogens (a cancer causing toxin) contribute to weight gain. Plus an added bonus is fiber makes you feel fuller longer decreasing cravings for the wrong types of foods.

Vitamins and minerals along with fiber help normalize hormones that can decrease cravings as well as plays a part in metabolism. For instance B vitamins play a role in fat, carbohydrate, protein breakdown and synthesis that contributes to our metabolism. Our metabolism influences how easily our bodies gain or lose weight. There are 8 B vitamins that are essential to our diet on a daily basis. These 8 B vitamins play a role in energy metabolism, grains such as wheat contains all of them in the kernel form-unprocessed.

However, the food refinement industry strips the kernel until all that's left is the endosperm which is basically a high starch carbohydrate. Once the refinement is complete and it has been turned into your favorite food such as bread, by law, the manufacturer adds back 4 synthetic versions of B vitamins; B1, B2, B3 and B9. B vitamins work synergistically and all are needed in order to work in the body properly. B vitamins work on not only energy metabolism but the metabolism and utilization of fatty acids, carbohydrates and protein synthesis. If you are not breaking down your nutrients this can lead to weight gain and fat accumulation especially in the abdominal area.

4) Are there any foods and products people who want to promote healthy weight should altogether avoid?

I won't name any products specifically however, in my opinion avoiding products with ingredients you cannot pronounce or recognize is a wise choice and something I share with my clients. Most of the ingredients found in

processed refined foods have detrimental consequences to health. There are thousands of food additives allowed by the FDA in our food. A 2013 study found that almost 80% of allowed food additives lack a level of safe consumption and 93% of food additives lack reproductive or developmental toxicity data.http://www.sciencedirect.com/science/article/pii/S 0890623813003298 In other words, we are the lab rats!

Monosodium glutamate (MSG) is an excitotoxin used to make bland foods taste better. MSG has been shown to kill sensitive neurons in the brain that can regulate appetite. Numerous studies indicate those who consume

MSG products are more likely to be overweight or obese. One study found men and women who ate the most MSG (a median of 5 grams a day) were about 30 percent more likely to become overweight by the end of the study than those who ate the least amount of the flavoring (less than a half-gram a day), http://ajcn.nutrition.org/content/93/6/1328 MSG has also been linked to obesity, eye damage, headaches, fatigue, depression and rapid heartbeat.

Synthetic sweeteners such as Aspartame, acesulfame-K (also known as acesulfame potassium or Ace-K) found in products such as candy, drinks, chewing gum and anything else that is "sugar free" or say "no sugar added." It has been approved by the U.S. Food and Drug Administration (FDA) as a food additive since 1988. According to the Yale Journal of Biology and Medicine has found a rise in the percent of the population who are obese coincides with an increase in the widespread use of non-caloric artificial sweeteners, such as aspartame and, research studies suggest that artificial sweeteners may contribute to weight gain. The study cites several large scale cohort studies finding positive correlations between artificial sweetener use and weight gain. **http://www.ncbi.nlm.nih.gov/pmc/articles/PMC28 92765/**

Why this leads to weight gain? Our hormones play a huge role in making us feel full and also control energy and fat storage. Two amino acids phenylalanine and aspartic acid found in aspartame stimulate the release of insulin and leptin two primary hormones that regulate metabolism and are involved in fat storage and satiety. Consuming aspartame products leads to increased levels of circulating lepton and insulin turning off the hormonal signal to stop eating and burning fat. You are eating like crazy to satisfy your cravings (usually empty caloric high sugar type foods) and your body responds by storing the excess energy as fat. This leads to inulin and leptin resistance essentially turning you from an energy burner to a fat storage machine!

Emulsifiers are added to foods to thicken or make them creamy. One study mouse showed that in comparison to control mice, previously healthy mice that were fed emulsifiers had low-level gastrointestinal inflammation, ate more food and gained more weight (especially body fat), had higher blood sugar levels and were resistant to the action of insulin. http://www.nature.com/ni/journal/v16/n4/full/ni.3103.html The mice were displaying evidence of metabolic syndrome. Metabolic syndrome is characterized by excessive abdominal fat, high blood pressure, increased levels of "bad" LDL-cholesterol and reduced levels of "good" HDL-cholesterol, poor blood sugar and an increased risk of type 2 diabetes, heart disease and stroke.

Avoid food ingredients such as these listed below:

- Soya Lecithin Granules G
- Soya Lecithin Powder P
- (Ultralec® P & G)
- Soya Lecithin Liquid (Yelkin® TS)
- Soya Lesithin-Powder,Granulate,Liquid
- Distilled Glycerin Monostearate(D...
- Potassium Stearate
- Calcium Stearoyl Lactylate(CSL)
- DATEM
- Mono and Diglycerides
- Glyceryl Monostearate
- Mono Propylene Glycol
- SPAN 80
- Sodium stearoyl lactylate(SSL)
- Tween
- Sodium Stearate
- Glycerol Triacetate
- Sugar Esters
- Polyglycerol Esters of Fatty Acid...
- Non dairy creamer
- Calcium Stearate
- Polyglycerol Polyricinoleate (PGPR)
- E No: E476
  http://www.chemistryindustry.biz/emulsifiers.html

5) Does someone have to starve to lose weight?

No you do not have to starve to lose weight. In fact eating more of the right foods throughout the day along with when you eat will lead to greater weight loss than starving. Diets of the past had us starving known as crash diets. The problem with chronic dieters using the starvation method leads to greater weight gain when the dieting period is over.

This is known as "feast and famine" syndrome. When we starve ourselves our body will used stored fat for energy. We lose the weight and then eat normally. Because the body knows that this is a regular occurrence will switch into "feast" mode and store the food you bring in as fat in anticipation for the next "famine" or diet period. You not only gain all the weight back but also end up gaining more weight then what you started.

The smart way to lose weight is to change your perception to food and diets. It is better to change to a healthier lifestyle that includes the right foods so that you can continuously maintain the weight you desire. Eating foods that are high in good fats and protein and keeping refined carbohydrates to a minimum allows for balanced insulin and balanced blood sugar thus reducing cravings. Fat is highly satiating and turns off our cravings for sugar. Fats also increase our metabolism to burn off excess thus leading to desired weight maintenance.

Eating throughout the day, starting with a good high protein, high fat breakfast will decrease cravings that happen later in the day. Basically it regulates blood sugar thus reducing cravings leading to less food intake and better intake of foods that work with metabolism instead of against it.

6) What is the best way to address appetite when making dietary changes?

Chewing. So simple and yet we do not do it enough. Chewing mixes our food with saliva mixed with enzymes that break down our food for better absorption later in the intestinal tract. Chewing also triggers the stomach for incoming food thus expanding the stomach. Chewing food 25-50 times before swallowing will allow sufficient time for expansion and decreases appetite thus eating less leading to weight loss.

Start with eating the right fats such as nuts, seeds, coconut, avocado, and oils much as olive oil and flax seed oil. The more fat you put into your diet the more full and satisfied you will feel. One study found that unsaturated fatty acids promote satiety which will help the body to establish energy balance. One study, found that subjects gained significantly more energy after consumption of lunch containing saturated fat than after the lunches containing either mono or polyunsaturated fat; additionally, there was a trend that these effects would continue into the next day. Lawton et al. (2000) http://www.ncbi.nlm.nih.gov/books/NBK53552/#ch14.r74

7) What causes cravings? Mental? Physical? Both?

There are many reasons for cravings from emotions to physical. One of the reasons we have a craving mechanism is to attract to us the foods that we need to correct a possible nutrient deficiency. For instance in the 18th century when sailors were ravaged with scurvy, they were also plagued with intense craving for fruits and vegetables. Scurvy is a disease caused by a diet lacking vitamin C. Ascorbic acid another word for vitamin C is found in citrus fruits as well as papaya, pineapple, kiwifruit, strawberries, cantaloupe along with broccoli, bell peppers, Brussel sprouts and cauliflower. In the 1800's there was not a lot of attention devoted to researching vitamins and minerals. To end the suffering of the sailors, researchers tried different sets of substances to help the sailors and it was limes that reversed the disease. Limes are a great source of vitamin C.

A 1939 study in which a group of toddlers were put in charge of feeding themselves, they were offered 34 nutritionally diverse whole foods, including water, potatoes, beef, bone jelly, carrots, chicken, grains, bananas and milk. What each child ate, and how much, was entirely up to him or her. According to the study, the toddlers were drawn to the foods that best nourished them. They ate more protein during growth spurts and more carbs and fat during periods of peak activity. After an outbreak of mononucleosis, curiously, they consumed more raw beef, carrots and beets. One child with a severe vitamin D deficiency drank cod liver

oil until he was cured.
http://www.ncbi.nlm.nih.gov/pmc/articles/PMC1626509/

We innately crave the foods we need to maintain balance in our body which usually consists of whole foods including live stock. Unfortunately, the refinement industry also knows that we are innately attracted to colorful fruits and vegetables and send millions of dollars on packing to attract us to their products. Our taste buds, along with our intuition, are highly confused. We rely on the color help with our deficiency instead we are rewarded with highly addictive substances that keep us continually eating trying to satiate the deficiency.

There is also the emotional cravings that we try to satiate with food. Part of what I teach is the emotional connections to food and what they mean. For instance, fat fried foods are to satiate the longing to fill up the emptiness we feel inside. Chocolate is about love, sensuality and longing to connect with our spiritual self. Nuts and nut butter are our longing for fun. Dairy products are considered antidepressants.

One of my clients was addicted to Rocky Road ice cream. Her freezer was filled with cartons of Rocky Road ice-cream, and she had coupons clipped for every store to get it on sale. As a Somatic Intuitive Trainer, I help people with their emotional connections to food. In one of our sessions, Elaine was extremely giddy and could not stop talking about her favorite ice cream. I had Elaine (name changed) close her eyes and imagine she was eating her ice cream. As I observed, her she was really experiencing the ice cream; she was smiling and looked like she was enjoying every imaginary bite.

After a while, I asked her to look beyond her ice cream. Her face changed. She became sad; it looked as if the color drained from her face. She saw her mother who was dying in the hospital. She was too late to say anything to her.

I guided her through and had her tell her mother what she longed to say. In that moment came clarity. Her truth had been said and days after (to this day) she no longer craves Rocky Road ice cream. Elaine's depression was in her inability to make her situation right by her. She felt depressed (dairy) not being able to say to say goodbye to her mother. Because of this she felt she could not be loved (chocolate) and enjoy her life (nuts).

Interesting to note, dairy products contain caseomorphins; opiate compounds that looks chemically the same as morphine found in cow's milk to slightly addict the calf to drink and allow for bonding. Cheese and chocolate contain small quantities of the neurotransmitter anandamide, an endogenous cannabinoid found in the brain. Anandamide targets the same brain structures as THC, the active ingredient in cannabis. Another neurotransmitter phenylethylamine stimulates the brain's pleasure centers promoting expressions of attraction, excitement, giddiness and, if over stimulated apprehension.

As you can see cravings are complex. There is the emotional need, nutritional need as well as the physical need that impacts our cravings.

8) How do you break the sugar addiction?

Balance blood sugar first. Of course, this means eating foods that are not high in sugar. Swap out refined sugary products for the whole food counter parts. For instance, if you drink orange juice in the morning, switch it out for a whole orange. Orange juice is literally liquid sugar. This goes right in to the blood stream spiking the production of insulin and leads to much quicker blood sugar spikes. In a couple of hours, blood sugar will drastically drop leading to cravings for carbohydrates or sugar. An orange on the other hand has all of its pulp. The fibrous pulp slows down the orange juice and allows for more stable blood sugar thus, reducing cravings later in the day. Better yet, take the whole peeled orange, add a handful of spinach and a good protein powder with a quarter avocado and blend in a blender to make a shake that will give you natural energy substance that will balance blood sugar.

9) Do you think parasites like Candida can contribute to difficult weight loss?

We are supposed to have hundreds of species of microscopic bacteria known as microbiota in our intestinal tract. Their role is to work in harmony with our immune system, digest food, and protect us against pathogenic and opportunistic bacteria and maintain our weight. Microbiota also create and allow for the absorption of vitamins such as B12 and vitamin K2 and minerals such as magnesium.

When there is an imbalance this can lead to cravings for the wrong types of foods to satiate the chemical messengers of the opportunistic bacteria.

A recent study took a group of Africans who ate a traditional local diet high in beans and vegetables and swapped their diet with a group of African Americans who ate a diet high in fat and animal proteins and low dietary fiber. In just two weeks, the African groups metabolism changed to an unhealthy profile including a pre-diabetes suggestion. http://journals.plos.org/plosone/article?id=10.1371/journal.pone.0035240

Our microbiota are highly adaptive to our internal and external conditions. As we change our food our bacteria changes to allow for the right strains to be in place to break down the incoming food. If we are eating a healthy diet full of fibers vegetables and other whole foods bacteria will create butyric acid which are short-chain-fatty-acids. Once absorbed into our bloodstream, these fatty acids can positively influence health by reducing our appetite and lowering our blood sugar levels. Butyrate and acetate were reported to protect against diet-induced obesity

Candida, a type of yeast, can cause stubborn fat deposits that are hard to lose leading to difficulties in losing weight. Candida feeds off of sugar in order to proliferate and to grow. We all have candida in our body; however, it is in healthy numbers when there is a good source of other bacteria such as saccharomyces boulardii that keep them in check. When the conditions allow for opportunistic yeast to grow, they quickly crowd at other bacteria and take over. To do this they require large amounts of sugar. They eat the sugar in your blood stream triggering your body to think it has low blood sugar thus signaling your body to eat more carbohydrates and sugar. Candida also creates up to 80 different toxins. Over time as the candida grows more and more toxins are dumped into the blood stream and overwhelming the liver. The liver is already busy creating bile, distributing nutrients and detoxifying harmful toxins. With the influx of candida the liver cannot deal with the burden and sends the toxins into fat cells usually in the abdominal area.

10) Why do you believe the current culture in the US is plagued with yo-yo dieting?

We learn through observation. We do what our parents do. Think about what you share? We share food and behavior. So, if you were a part of a family who tried every diet without success, most will follow the same behavior. We also eat the foods that our family ate. We learn our basic nutrition philosophy through our parents. We are bombarded with messages in our print material, television ads, and we are tracked through cookies on our social media sites. We are constantly, sublimely told what is good and not good for us. Weight loss industries know our trigger pain points and market the next pharmaceutical to aid in weightless by emotionally connecting with us.

11) How do you coach your clients to break the cycle of serial dieting?

The first thing I do when I work with a client is instruct them to weigh themselves, record it and take the scale and hide it! We are fixated on a scale and yet weight fluctuates on a daily basis. Instead I have them focus on how their clothes fit and how they feel. If the clothes feel loose then they are losing weight and, this also more rewarding than a fluctuating scale!

I work with them as a whole taking into consideration their lifestyle, the family dynamics, their emotional health. I take this information and educate them on how dieting is not the answer rather lifestyle change.

I empower them to try something new that is going to become a habit. So, choose one thing, master it and then add something else. This sets them up for success. I also work on increasing fats, protein and whole vegetables along with while reducing carbohydrates. I do not believe in cheat days because it sounds like they are eating forbidden foods on days that don't count! Every day counts! We are not on a diet but a lifelong healthy journey. I teach them how to make deserts from coconut and nut flour such as almond flour that are a part of a healthy diet that can be enjoyed every day. It is really about changing language and seeing their diet in a new light that makes the biggest impact.

I work on changing their gut microbiota to one that is going to work for them. I have them take specific human microflora strains as well as clean up any leaky gut, remove inflammatory foods that lead to weigh gain and bloating, and get their digestion system working optimally so that they can break down the nutrients from their diet and utilize to help maintain weight. The question I get from clients most often that follow my program is "Karen how do I stop losing weight?"

Now that is music to my ears!

MELISSA'S TIPS & TRICKS

People often ask what diet and exercise programs did I use to lose my weight; honestly, my philosophy follows more of a whole health focus that boils down to the following guidelines:

1) Drink daily your weight in ounces of water.
(Hydration curbs hunger.)

2) Drink water with lemons or lemon essential oil.
(Assists with detoxification)

3) Don't skip meals. Carry protein shakes if necessary.
(Keeps hunger under control)

4) Eat a source of protein with every meal and snack.
(Helps regulate blood sugar and slows the digestion of carbs)

5) Eat carb rich foods earlier in the day and finish the day with proteins and veggies

6) Try to eat alkaline foods as much as possible.
(Green leafy veggies, high in nutrition with disease/cancer fighting properties)

7) Avoid processed foods or items with more than 5 ingredients
(Know what you are consuming)

8) Eat organic produce as much as knowingly possible
(Minimize consumption of toxins, wash ALL produce)

9) Take organic supplements to avoid vitamin deficiencies.

10) Walk, a lot. I do a minimum of 60 minutes every day.
(Add other activities as desired in addition to walking).

HELPFUL LINKS

Visit my website for more resources such as : Blog Posts, Links to Social Media Pages, Information about Webinars and Public appearances, Promotions and Contests.

www.fromplussizetopinup.com

NUTRITION:
http://PlusSizetoPinup.le-vel.com

ESSENTIAL OILS:
www.mydoterra.com/melissaglossup

ABOUT THE AUTHOR

Melissa Michelle Glossup, MA., M.Ed. struggled with her weight her entire life. When she was 16, her family enrolled her in a program called Metabolic Research Center. Through this program, she lost 60 lbs., could wear a size 6, and represented her hometown Abilene, Texas in the Miss National Teenage America Pageant West Texas. At 18, her family could no longer afford the program, and she stopped taking the supplements in February of 1998. By May, she had gained 80 lbs. From there, she continued to gain around 40 pounds a year until she reached a staggering 375+ lbs.

In 2008, she changed her thoughts, she changed her body, she changed her life. Over the past few years, she shed and maintained a weight loss exceeding 225 lbs.

Melissa's vision is to raise awareness and advocate funding to establish educational healthy lifestyle programs and develop curriculums to prevent childhood obesity.

Melissa has a Masters of Arts in English, a Masters of Arts in Linguistics, a Masters of Secondary Education, and an esteemed faculty member at the University of Phoenix.